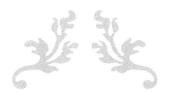

EMOTIONAL INTELLIGENCE

A Complete Beginners Guide To Become The Leader That Everyone Likes And Boost Your Work Performance By Positive Psychology. Develop The Leader Within You, And Increase Your Self Confidence

DALE ECKHART

Legal & Disclaimer

The information contained in this book and its contents is not designed to replace or take the place of any form of medical or professional advice; and is not meant to replace the need for independent medical, financial, legal or other professional advice or services, as may be required. The content and information in this book has been provided for educational and entertainment purposes only.

The content and information contained in this book has been compiled from sources deemed reliable, and it is accurate to the best of the Author's knowledge, information and belief. However, the Author cannot guarantee its accuracy and validity and cannot be held liable for any errors and/or omissions. Further, changes are periodically made to this book as and when needed. Where appropriate and/or necessary, you must consult a professional (including but not limited to your doctor, attorney, financial advisor or such other professional advisor) before using any of the suggested remedies, techniques, or information in this book.

Upon using the contents and information contained in this book, you agree to hold harmless the Author from and against any damages, costs, and expenses, including any legal fees potentially resulting from the application of any of the information provided by this book. This disclaimer applies to any loss, damages or injury caused by the use and application, whether directly or

Table of Contents

INTRODUCTION

If you are currently reading this, it means you are one of the people striving so hard to get rid of anger, stress, and anxiety in order to build a life of positivity for themselves. Well, count yourself lucky because you have just found your one-stop-shop to everything you need to know about anger, stress, and anxiety management; you can now find out everything you need to know about overcoming negativity. The book, "Master your Emotions" contains genuine information, tips, strategies, and techniques that can help you create that happy, negativity-devoid, and quality life you desire and as well, deserve. The book is written in simplified and easy-to-digest language to help you assimilate everything contained within smoothly.

The book will teach you all you need to know about stress management, anxiety management, and anger management by making you privy to some of the most effective techniques and strategies for mastering your emotions and learning emotional intelligence. This book will begin by explaining all the basics you need to know about emotions; the nature of emotions; and the sources of emotions. What impacts our emotions? How are emotions developed? Are negative emotions even necessary at all? How can you get rid of them? These and many more are the questions you will be finding valid answers to in "Master your emotions: improve your emotional intelligence by controlling your mind and boost your brain to eliminate your anxiety and worry."

We will also take an in-depth look at what emotional intelligence is and how it can help you rid your life of negativity. Most importantly, you will learn about anger management and core relaxation strategies to get rid of worries, concerns, and uncertainties. To further help you, we will be giving you tips on how to practice mindfulness meditation which is a popular form of meditation now being used to practice self-awareness. Mindfulness meditation technique can help you develop your connection with your inner self so that you can develop high emotional intelligence.

If you are interested in leading a value-laden life, qualitative, and filled with positivity; if you want to learn to project positivity into negative emotions and you would like to learn how you can be more productive, purposeful, and positive in life but you don't know where to begin from, this one-stop-shop for positivity promises to teach you these and everything else you need to know. Every answer you need awaits you in this amazing read.

The choice is now left to you to choose a life devoid of stress, anger, anxiety; a life of positivity; and start living life with a de-cluttered and free mind using the strategies, tips, and techniques waiting for you in the book. Add a copy to the cart and get started on the journey to positivity and productivity!

However, it wasn't until 1995, when Daniel Goleman published his book by the same name, that emotional intelligence rolled into the mainstream consciousness and became a ground-breaking concept. Back then, intelligence quotient was seen as the only factor that mattered when it came to assessing an individual's capabilities. Once emotional intelligence took over, IQ was perceived as a narrow or limited way of assessing an individual's chances of success. The cut-throat world of career, jobs, and business was starkly different from the cushy confines of a classroom.

If one had to navigate the real world, they'd have to adapt to a different kind of intelligence than the academic one used in classrooms or libraries. A person's knowledge and cognitive abilities alone didn't guarantee success in life. A degree didn't automatically mean a high paying job or a profitable business.

At best, you'll get your foot through the door. However, for someone to succeed, you would need much more than just plain intelligence. It would take social, communication, conversation, and emotional skills to raise the bar. These are life skills that don't come in the classroom but are learned by living in a hostel, waiting at bars, joining social clubs, being a part of sports teams, and volunteering.

CHAPTER 1:WHAT ARE EMOTIONS

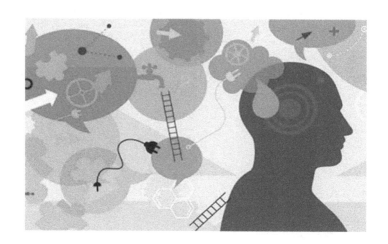

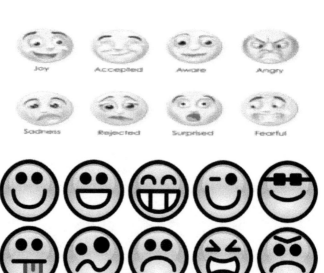

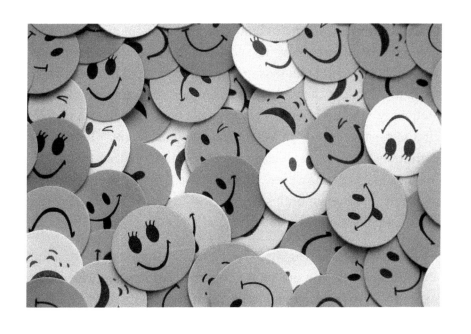

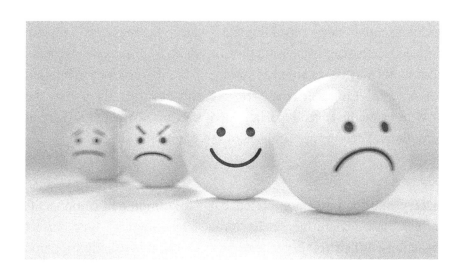

Understanding the nature of emotions and what emotions are is the first step to learning how to successfully master your emotions. After all, how could you master something if you don't even know what it is or how it works? In a simpler definition, the Oxford dictionary says emotion is "a strong feeling deriving from one's circumstances, mood, or relationships with others." From both definitions, you can already tell that emotions are related to feelings in a way. However, emotions and feelings are not entirely the same. Human emotions are usually triggered by changes in a person's physiological and behavioral makeup.

As humans, we can usually tell our emotional state at every point. You know when you are feeling happy, sad, or angry. However, what you probably cannot tell is where exactly these feelings originate from. Usually, most of us make the mistake of regarding emotions and feelings as the same thing. We even use both interchangeably in the form of synonyms. But, like we have said; emotions and feelings are two different things that are somewhat dependent on each other. While emotions originate from a subconscious and physiological state, feelings are mostly subjective to experiences and they originate from a conscious state. Emotions may be regarded as automatic bodily reactions to internal or external triggers. Therefore, we can say that there may be emotions without feelings but there can be no feelings without emotions. Feelings are subjects of our emotional state.

Types of emotions

Every emotion humans experience has four important components which are: cognitive, behavioral, physiological, and affect reactions. When you experience an emotion, it is usually triggered and fueled by any of these four components.

Firstly, cognitive reaction to emotions refers to how a person thinks, stores information and experiences, and perceives an event. Behavioral reactions have to do with how humans primarily express an emotion. Physiological reactions on the other hand are triggered by changes in a person's hormonal level. Finally, affect reactions signify the state of emotion and the nature of the emotion itself. Each aspect of emotions as explained usually triggers the other. For instance, let's say that an aunt you don't like comes to visit your parents; immediately you see this person, you automatically think in your mind that she is annoying or scary probably due to past experiences with her and her disposition (this is a cognitive reaction). Due to this perception you have of your annoying aunt, you become grumpy (this is the affect reaction). Then, your parents come to tell you that your aunt will be staying in the house for a while; you feel your blood rising in anger (this is a physiological reaction) and you angrily leave for your room (behavioral reaction). To understand the different components of emotions, you must ensure you know where emotions originate from. Experts have tried to identify the source of emotions using different theories. These theories try to explain the processes of emotions formulation, the sources of emotions, and the cause. We will be looking into these theories, although not in-depth. We will try to understand how emotions occur solitarily.

In the bid to explain emotions, researchers have formulated different theories which are classified under three main categories. We have the physiological theories which propose that emotions are the results of certain responses within the body; there are the neurological theories which suggest that certain activities that take place in the brain are responsible for our emotions; finally, there are theories under the cognitive class which believe that our thoughts, perceptions, and mental activities are responsible for the formulation of emotions.

The first theory that tries to explain emotions is the "evolutionary theory of emotion" which was proposed by Charles Darwin, a naturalist. This theory argues that emotions evolve due to their adaptive nature which promotes human survival and reproduction. Darwin also said that humans seek to reproduce with mates due to feelings of love and affection which are products of emotions. He further explained that feelings of fear cause people to recognize and flee from danger. According to Darwin, we have emotions because we need them to adapt and survive in whatever environment we find ourselves. Emotions trigger appropriate responses to certain stimuli in the environment, thereby promoting our chances of survival. To survive in any environment, we have to be cognizant of our own emotions and that of others. However, it is not enough to be aware of emotions, we must also be able to interpret, control, and respond appropriately to a trigger. Being able to correctly interpret our emotions and that of others makes it possible for us to give suitable and appropriate responses to any situation we find ourselves.

Next is the James-Lange theory which is a prominent physiological theory of emotion. This theory was proposed individually by Carl Lange, a physiologist, and William James, a psychologist. The James-Lange theory of emotion argues that emotions are bodily responses which are triggered as a result of the body's physiological reactions to certain events. According to James and Lange, the emotions you produce in response to a physiological reaction caused by a stimuli in the environment is dependent on your interpretation of the physiological reaction. For instance, if you are watching a frightening scene in a movie and you feel your heart start to race, James and Lange believe that you will interpret

15

the physiological reaction (of your heart racing) as you being scared. Then, you conclude that you are frightened since your heart is racing. The James-Lange physiological theory of emotion proposes that your heart isn't racing because you are scared; rather, you are scared because your heart is racing. Therefore, the emotion of fear you are feeling at that point in time is a response to the physiological reaction taking place in your body.

Another prominent theory which seeks to explain the origin and nature of emotions is the Cannon-Bard theory of emotion. This is also a physiological theory but it seeks to directly counter the submissions of James and Lange. Proposed by Walter Cannon and further expanded by Philip Bard, this theory explains that humans experience physiological reactions linked to certain emotions without necessarily experiencing these emotions. For example, your heart also races when you do something exciting such as exercise, not just when you are scared. According to Cannon, people experience emotional responses so quickly that they simply can't be the results of some physical reactions. As an example, when you watch that frightening movie scene, you often start to feel scared even before noticing that your heart is racing or your hands are trembling. Cannon and Bard, in essence, argue that emotional responses and physiological reactions often occur simultaneously to internal or external stimuli.

The Schechter-Singer theory is another theory of emotion which examines emotions from a cognitive perspective. According to this theory, humans first experience a physiological reaction after which they try to identify the cause of this reaction so they can experience it as an emotion. In other words, you react to external or internal stimuli with a physiological response which you then interpret from a cognitive perspective; the result of the cognitive interpretation is what is considered an emotion. The Schechter and

16

Singer theory is quite similar to both James-Lange and Cannon-Bard theory but the main difference is the cognitive interpretation which humans use to label an emotion, according to Schechter and Singer. Like Cannon and Bard, Schechter and Singer also argued that certain physiological responses in the body can result in different emotions.

The Lazarus theory of emotion or Cognitive Appraisal theory as it is also called was proposed by Richard Lazarus and is another theory that takes a cognitive approach. This theory suggests that thinking always takes place before emotion is experienced. According to Lazarus and other pioneers of this theory, humans react to stimuli immediately with thoughts, after which the physiological response and emotions are experienced. This means that your thoughts always come first before a physiological and emotional response. For example, if you are watching a frightening scene in a movie, your mind immediately starts to think that this movie is scary and frightening. This triggers an emotion of fear, accompanied by related physical reactions such as hands trembling, racing heart, etc.

Finally, we have the Facial-Feedback theory of emotion. This theory suggests that emotional experiences are linked to our facial expressions. What this means is that your physical reactions to stimuli have a direct impact on the emotion you experience, instead of being the effects of the emotion. This theory argues that our emotions are directly linked to changes in our facial muscles. For instance, if you force yourself to smile more when interacting with people, you will have a better time at social events. And, if you carry a frown whenever you interact with people at social events, you'd definitely feel an awful emotion.

These are all theories of emotions which experts have proposed over the years. You may wonder why you even need to learn about the theories of emotions just because you want to learn how to control your emotions. To master your emotions, there is one key thing you must first do; understand how emotions occur. If you want to learn to control an emotion like anger, you definitely need to first identify the source of the anger and all the symptoms associated with it. Once you know this, you can easily put a leash on your rage the next time you feel it brewing.

Emotions are an important part of our lives because they have huge impacts on our actions, reactions, decisions, and ultimately, our lives. There may still be a huge cloud of mystery surrounding why humans experience emotions but with the little knowledge available to us, we should be able to understand and manage our emotions effectively.

Anger

Anger is one of the most unwanted emotions, yet it is frequently manifested. One of the causes of anger is when an individual feels entitled to something. For instance, if you feel that you deserve an award, respect, and attention, then you are on the path of attracting anger when you get disappointment. Most people that tend to be temperamental also show low self-esteem suggesting that each disappointment they get makes them think they are destined to be failures. If unmanaged, anger can cost your health, social life, work, and finances.

Fear/Discomfort

Whenever we try something new, we experience anxiety. We are afraid of the unknown. This is why we like to maintain our daily routine and stay within our comfort zones. From our brain's point of view, this makes perfect sense. If our current habits allow us to be safe and avoid any potential threat to our survival (or the survival of our ego) why bother changing them? This explains why we often keep the same routine or have the same thoughts over and over. It is also why we may experience a lot of internal resistance when trying to change ourselves.

Grief

It is important to grieve the loss of someone or something important in your life, but grief can snowball into a debilitating emotion if it isn't managed correctly. If you find yourself overwhelmed by grief, try to be more active. It is easy while grieving to withdraw socially and stop doing productive activities. Force yourself to engage with others and seek the emotional support that you need from the people you are close to. Don't let your life stagnate. Keep practicing mindfulness, exercising, eating right, and everything else that makes you feel good.

Understand that you don't have to feel guilty for moving on from a loss. Just because you have accepted the loss of that thing or person doesn't mean you've forgotten.

Happiness

As one of the most sought after feelings, happiness regards what we wish to feel in an appealing manner. There are numerous efforts and strategies at personal, community, and governmental levels to enhance levels of happiness as it directly impacts the health of people. Happiness, as an emotion, is manifested through body languages such as a relaxed stance, facial expressions like smiling, and an upbeat illustrated by a pleasant tone of voice.

Like any other emotion, the emotion of happiness is largely created by human experience and the belief system. For instance, if scoring sixty marks is regarded as desirable, then a student is likely to feel happy to attain or surpass the mark. If riding in a train with family members is regarded as being happy then an individual that never had that experience might feel happy and eager at the prospect of boarding a train. Fortunately, we can optimize happiness by enhancing our emotional intelligence levels.

Sadness

As an emotion, sadness is a transient emotional state whose attributes include hopelessness, grief, disappointment, dampened mood, and disinterest. There are several ways to manifest sadness as emotion, and these include:

- **Withdrawal from others**
- **Dampened mood**
- **Lethargy**
- **Crying**
- **Quietness**

Envy

Envy commonly happens at the workplace where an employee admires to be accomplished just like the popular colleague. A human entertains and pursues ambitions routinely, and this allowed. The problem starts when one becomes uneasy with the accomplishments of others to the point of being affected mentally and physically; the person is feeling envious. As expected, persons with a feeling of envy will rarely acknowledge that they are manifesting the negative emotion. At the workplace, envy affects an individual negatively. While the limited and occasional form of envy is necessary to spur one to improve and strive for more, it becomes a problem if it is not managed. Feelings of envy are likely to commonly manifest at the workplace as workplaces appraise employees and reward those accomplished ones.

Overcoming envy requires accepting that we have different competencies and different timings. By accepting that there are individuals more qualified than you will help you create room for accepting others to become more successful than you. It is also important to observe that seasoned employees are likely to deliver compared to recruits. Ability to unlearn can help in managing the feeling of envy. As with any emotion, it is not possible to escape from feeling envy, but one can effectively manage the feeling. When the feeling of envy sets in, convince yourself that in one hour, you will shed off that feeling and not react to the accomplishment of a friend or colleague.

Anxiety

Feeling worried is important to enabling one to visualize and plan for the worst-case scenarios. For instance, being worried about passing exams enables you to address the risk of failing by working harder, consulting, or planning for failure as a possible outcome of the test that you took. However, worry becomes a bad emotion when it takes over you and prevents one from routine activities and routine interactions. For instance, when you constantly feel worried about failure making you study until you get burnout then worry as emotion becomes a negative emotion. As earlier on indicated, feelings emanate from human experience and system of beliefs, and this implies that if the society does not accommodate failure, then you will get the emotion of worry. The emotion is manifesting because of past experiences and the current system of beliefs regarding exams and not necessarily about how you feel internally.

Self-criticism

Self-judgment happens when we critic ourselves and found ourselves inadequate. Self-criticism is necessary as a way of self-evaluation and can help one improve performance, social skills, and communication. A fortunate aspect of human beings is that they can reflect over their experiences, detach from their self and evaluate themselves, and speak to oneself. Limited self-judgment can help increase personal accountability, which can increase the professionalism and appeal of an individual at the workplace and in society. However, self-criticism becomes an issue when one gets stuck at it and feels worthless before society.

Frustration

This is when you feel trapped but can't do anything about it. Frustration in the workplace is the most common cause of burnout.

Worry

With so many layoffs, it's natural to be worried about losing your job. However, instead of feeling anxious, try to focus on your job and think about ways of improving your performance, to you make yourself more employable. Nervous people usually have low self-confidence.

Disappointment

Repeated disappointments always negatively affect efficiency and productivity, and if unaddressed, can lead to burnout and high staff turnover.

The key thing about nurturing negative emotions in the workplace be it feelings about your colleagues, management, working environment, salary, or something else is that these feelings are contagious, and this kind of resentment easily spreads and demoralizes others. This is why a negative person is more likely to be fired, if for no other reason than to prevent their negativity and resentment from spreading to others.

Anger is often perceived from the point of a primary emotion but anger may also be a secondary emotion. In fact, anger is often more secondary than primary. Anger is a basic human emotion that is connected with our survival as humans. It is as basic as happiness, sadness, fear, and other elemental emotions. Like stress and anxiety, anger is also connected with the "fight or flight" response of the nervous system; it is meant for your protection and survival. The fight or flight response is usually activated when someone perceives danger; it prepares you to either fight or flee from the perceived danger. However, fighting in this response has evolved from actual fighting to other things. There are situations where "fighting" doesn't mean getting your punch ready; it may be reacting to an injustice by championing a cause for justice.

Contrary to what you have been made to believe, anger is a perfectly normal, usually healthy, and natural human emotion. But, anger can also become destructive when it gets out of control. We all feel anger at some point in time although in varying degree. This is due to the fact that anger is a part of our experiences as humans. Anger usually arises in varying context and is usually preceded by some emotion which could be pain, injustice, dissatisfaction, criticism, and unfairness generally. Usually, anger comes in different range from irritation to rage. Anger in the form of mild irritation may be caused by feelings of stress, tiredness, and anxiety. In fact, humans are likely to become irritated when their basic human needs like food, shelter, and sleep are not being met. We may also be irritated by thoughts and opinions from other people which do not conform to ours.

Often, when anger becomes an emotion we cannot control, it becomes destructive. It can have a massive impact on our personal and work relationship with others but it doesn't stop at this. Anger is also destructive to our health, physically and emotionally. With unchecked anger usually comes stress and when anger becomes prolonged, the stress hormones that come with anger can destroy certain neurons in some part of the brain responsible for short-term memory and judgment. Anger can also weaken the immune system.

As we have said, anger is a basic human emotion necessary for survival so there are times when anger can be positive and not "bad." In fact, anger is not really a "bad" emotion in itself; it becomes bad when we allow it get to us unchecked i.e. when it becomes uncontrollable. No emotion is necessarily bad as long as we are able to master and control these emotions. Anger may sometime be a substitute emotion which is being used to cover up for something like pain, envy, jealousy, etc. There are people who make themselves angry just so they don't have to feel pain. People change their emotions from pain to anger sometimes because it is easier to be angry than it is to be in pain. This may be a conscious or unconscious action.

Anger is usually grouped into several types by experts and for this book, we will be checking out 8 identified types of anger. Knowing the type or source of your anger makes it easier for this anger to be controlled or managed. All types of anger which we will be examining are psychologically based since anger is an emotion of the mind.

- **Righteous Anger:** This is a positive anger that we feel when an injustice has been committed or when we feel a rule has been broken. It may also be referred to as judgmental or moral anger because it is a morally indignant anger that may also arise due to our perception of someone else's shortcoming. This kind of anger usually stems from belief and rules. That anger you experience when you feel that someone's human right has been abused is a righteous anger. However, this sort of anger may assume a morally superior stance which is that you think you are better than some people and that is why you get angry with them; it may also be because you think someone is better than something they have done. Righteous anger may become excessive out of the need to manipulate and control others.

- **Assertive Anger:** Have you ever used your feelings of rage to initiate a social good or positive change? If yes, then this is what we refer to as assertive anger. It is a constructive kind of anger that serves as catalyst for initiating changes aimed at positively altering the state of something. Rather than express anger in form of confrontations, arguments, outbursts, and verbal abuse, people who get assertively angry express their rage in ways that create a positive change around the situation that got them angry in the first place. This is normally done without any form of destruction, distress, or anxiety. Assertive anger can be a really powerful motivator for you.

- **Aggressive Anger:** Also called behavioral anger, this type of anger is usually physically expressed. It is a highly volatile, unpredictable, and out-of-control that may push you to physically attack someone. But, this doesn't mean that this anger always results in harm or injuries. When this anger overwhelms you, it may push you to lash out at the object of your anger or something else nearby like the wall or a photo frame. Aggressive or behavioral anger may have huge legal and personal consequences. Trauma or neglect from childhood may be the root of this type of anger.

- **Habitual anger:** There are times when anger becomes a perpetual emotion due to the fact that you have spent so much time being angry. Habitual anger refers to when you are in a constant state of irritation, dissatisfaction, and unrest such that pretty much everything annoys you. People who have this kind of habitual anger may even get angrier when confronted about their anger or certain situations. The underlying secret behind this kind of anger is that it is always rooted deep in the past and it accumulates over the years probably due to negative experiences. The older you get without managing this anger, the more you feed it.

- **Chronic Anger:** This is a general and dangerous form of anger. It is the absolute and continual resentment of your situation, certain circumstances, people around you and even yourself. It is a form of habitual anger because it is also in perpetuity. Since it is a prolonged experience, chronic anger often have immensely adverse effects on an individual's mental and physical wellbeing.

- **Passive-Aggressive Anger:** People who try to avoid confrontations and expression of feelings are the ones who usually experience the passive-aggressive type of anger. Passive-aggressive anger has to do with repressing your anger, rage, or fury in order to avoid getting into arguments and confrontations. This kind of anger is often expressed subtly in the form of sarcasm, verbal abuse, mockery, veiled silence, and chronic procrastination. Most people who express anger passively often don't accept that they are aggressive but their actions may have damaging effects on their personal and professional relationship with others.

- **Verbal Anger:** Often, verbal anger is considered to be milder than aggressive or habitual anger but it is just as bad. This anger is a deeply emotional and psychological which has profound effects on the target of the abuse. It comes in form of threats, mockery, sarcasm, yelling, screaming, furious shouting, blaming, and poor criticism. It is often experienced out of annoyance or irritation.

- **Self-harm:** This is a kind of anger directed by oneself at oneself. It goes way beyond depression. For instance, there are people who cut themselves up; this could be them expressing anger because they probably don't like their looks. Self-harm is quite complicated however you should know that it is a very negative emotion which you can't hold in. Self-harm can be a result of so many thing; physical abuse, emotional abuse, neglect, and trauma. It may also be because of repeated disappointments. Rather than expressing their anger towards the person who has wronged them, some people focus the anger on their inner self.

No matter the type of anger you experience, there are some factors which are the major causes of anger. For effective anger management to take place, you must know and address the cause of your anger. So, let's check out some of the known causes of anger.

Factors that Contribute to Anger

There are many factors that contribute to why you get angry apart from the fact that anger is a natural emotion which you must experience. How you react to situations depend on certain factors in life and these factors are the ones that determine the degree of anger you experienced.

The first known factor that contributes how you experience anger is your childhood and upbringing. As children, many people have been taught certain beliefs about anger; they were taught that anger is destructive, bad, and very negative. Individuals who were taught that it is bad to express anger learn not to complain about injustice; they may have also been punished for expressing their anger as kids. So, they learn to keep the anger in till it becomes a long-term habitual problem. Sometimes, they end up expressing their anger in very unhealthy ways due to years of bottling all that emotions in. They may also turn the anger inwards if there are no other outlets. There are also people who have grown up thinking it is okay to be aggressive or violent so they tend to act out their anger aggressively. This may be because they weren't taught how to properly express their emotions or manage them.

Another factor that contributes to anger and how you react to situations is the past experiences you have had. As a child, if you have experienced situations which made you feel angry and resentful in the past but you weren't able to healthily express this anger at the time, you may still be nursing the anger till the present time. For instance, if you have been abused or you have faced trauma in the past, the anger may still be there lurking somewhere in your heart especially if you weren't able to do anything about it then. Of course, this results in you finding some situations particularly difficult and easy to get you angry.

Your anger problem may also be due to circumstances you are presently faced with and not just things you experienced in the past. Current circumstances and challenges may leave you feeling angrier than normal or make you get angry at things and situations that aren't even related. If there is a situation making you angry and you can't do anything about it, you may express the anger at other times under a totally different condition. As an example, if your boss at work makes you angry and stressed out every day but you can't do anything about it since he's your boss, you may express the anger at home rather than at work. For instance, you may get home and lash at the kids or your spouse grumpily or angrily and then blame it on a "long day."

These are 3 of the most influencing factors for what gets you angry and how you react to potentially raging situations.

Anger as a Positive Emotion

As much as we all like to consider anger a negative emotion, it can also be a positive emotion when we react to it the right way; it is also positive as long as we have our anger under control and never let it consume us. When anger is positive, it means it is driving us to do something beneficial; positive anger lays the foundation for changes and developments.

Positive anger is a highly motivating force which compels us to do something we may have thought we couldn't do in the past. Anger fuels our passion and drives us towards our goals no matter the challenges and barriers that seem to be in our way. It is a constructive kind of emotion which infuses us with the energy and motivation needed to get what we want; it can inspire a clamor for social change and justice (think Martin Luther King). Again, when anger is a positive emotion, it pushes us to be optimistic. Now, this may sound odd and impossible to you but it is true. Anger could make you optimistic just like happiness does.

Anger as a positive emotion can also be very beneficial to our relationships. It is a natural emotion and we have to strive to be as natural as possible in our relationships. There is no need to suck it in and repress your anger with a smile when your partner, relative, or friend wrongs you. According to research, anger becomes negative and detrimental to a relationship when you suppress or hide it. When you repress your anger and give a faux smile, you are not letting your partner know what they have done to wrong you so they may keep doing it which doesn't do the relationship good. However, when you express your anger positively and healthily, it strengthens your relationship and the bond you share with your partner. Anger helps you find solutions to whatever problem you have in your relationships.

Anger can also be positive when we use it for self-insight; this emotion is a pretty good tool for examining and looking inwards ourselves. Anger allows us to see our faults and work on them. If you never express your anger, there is every chance that you would never know what you doing wrong to people to get that reaction which triggers your anger. Sometimes, the fault is with you and not the person who made you angry. When you become self-conscious and self-aware, you can find ways through which you can channel your anger to improve your life for the better. Positive anger promotes positive self-change.

Okay, this next one sounds absolutely odd but what if you learned that anger reduces violence? Yes, it absolutely does. We all know that anger is an emotion that is known to precede violence so how can anger even reduce violence? What happens is that when you get angry, it may be a powerful pointer telling you that something needs to be changed or resolved. When you notice this, anger could motivate you to take actions to mediate the situation which could instigate violence if not checked. Take a moment and imagine a world where no one could react to injustice immediately with anger? Yeah, it does seem like a potentially violent world. Also, when someone wrongs us and we express our anger healthily, it may make them take actions to placate us and right the wrong they committed.

Finally, positive anger can be used to get what you want. One thing you should keep in mind at all time though is that anger can only be positively or used positively when it is justifiable. Anger which makes you feel control is not positive and cannot be used to initiate positive developments or changes. This is the kind of anger you'll need the anger management techniques we will be discussing for. Anger management techniques teach you to transform your anger from positive to negative.

Emotions and Your Mind

Your mind is unique. There is no other psychological framework like yours, and you will experience emotions differently than anyone else. Take falling in love as an example. This may feel like weightlessness/lightness, or it may feel as if a million bees are trapped inside your stomach. It may be intense, or it may be subtle. It may be instantaneous, or it may emerge gradually. It is the same with anger, frustration, weariness, and even happiness. Just because you may not experience the same emotion in the same way as another person does not devalue what you are experiencing.

Because no two people will experience the same emotion, in the same way, no definition will be appropriate for every person. For example, two people battling depression may experience very different symptoms. The first may have trouble sleeping, have no appetite, and have no interest in things that were once enjoyable while the second has trouble with sleeping in too long, binge-eating, and intense waves of despair. These two instances of depression will look strikingly different from an external viewer, but both of these sufferers' emotions and experiences are valid and could be identified as depression.

This is why intense emotions like grief affect different people in such disparate ways. Two siblings are facing the loss of a parent, for example, will each deal with it in his or her way. The first may cling to family and friends for support in coping with the intense grief, while the other may become the family comic, cracking jokes to keep everyone smiling while dealing with the sadness in private. Neither of these responses is wrong; they're just different.

The trick is to stop comparing your emotional self to the emotional selves of others. Identifying and defining emotions in one must be a personal affair. When we compare ourselves with others, we end up invalidating our feelings because they don't seem to "match what everyone else is feeling." Your emotions are yours, and they are valid already in the fact that you are experiencing them.

We do not experience every emotion at the same intensity every time, by which I mean emotional intensity, varies depending on what the experience is. For example, you may experience a low-intensity grief after hearing the news that a favorite performer has passed away, but you may experience a much fuller, more intense grief at the loss of a friend or relative.

As low-and mild-intensity emotions tend to be easier to cope with, these are often constructive. You may cry over the loss of that beloved celebrity, but these tears would likely be cathartic, granting inner relief through the expression of the emotion. A high-intensity emotion, on the other hand, can be more difficult to face or cope with, causing emotional and psychological distress. The loss of a friend, for example, may cause that much higher intensity of grief, making it difficult to continue with daily life.

Not everyone experiences emotions with the same intensity. Some of us are just designed to feel more intensely than others. If you've ever found yourself overcome with emotion over what was, for others, a mundane situation, then you may be an intense feeler. This is not a bad thing, because it also means you feel positive emotions more intensely, but being an intense feeler may be why you struggle with mismanaged emotions. The higher the intensity, the more difficult emotions can be to cope with.

Let's consider depression as an example. We all experience sadness at some point in our lives because we all deal with dissatisfaction and loss, but severe, high-intensity depression is a debilitating and dangerous emotion. It is natural and normal to become sad after a disappointment or a tragic event, but our general perceptions and thought patterns are typically not severely altered by it. We cope with temporary sadness and then move on with our lives. Depression is not so easy to overcome. It is a high-intensity emotion that can severely affect thoughts, feelings, and behaviors, sometimes without any identifiable trigger. Coping with sadness is a difficult but manageable chore while coping with depression is a long-term and complicated journey.

The Nature of Emotions

Emotions can be tricky. By understanding the mechanism behind emotions, you'll be able to manage them more effectively as they arise.

The first thing to understand is that emotions come and go. One moment you feel happy, the next you feel sad. While you do have some control over your emotions, you must also recognize their unpredictable nature. If you expect to be happy all the time, you set yourself up for failure. You then risk blaming yourself when you 'fail' to be happy, or even worse, beat yourself up for it.

To start taking control of your emotions, you must accept they are transient. You must learn to let them pass without feeling the need to identify strongly with them. You must allow yourself to feel sad without adding commentaries such as, "I shouldn't be sad," or "What's wrong with me?" Instead, you must allow reality to be.

Typically, when someone is described as emotional, this is intended to be taken in a negative light. Emotional people are often regarded as impulsive, difficult to talk to, difficult to work with, unscientific, irrational, loud, or resistant to being spoken to. But this characterization is based on assumptions about emotional people. Indeed, labeling someone as emotional is a simple and almost devious way to neutralize and invalidate someone by immediately labeling them as something which they may or may not be.

No matter how mentally tough you are, you'll still experience sadness, grief, or depression in your life hopefully not at the same time, and not continually. At times, you'll feel disappointed, betrayed, insecure, resentful, or ashamed. You'll doubt yourself and doubt your ability to be the person you want to be. But that's okay because emotions come, but, more importantly, they go.

CHAPTER 2: CONSTRUCTIVE EMOTIONS AND DESTRUCTIVE EMOTIONS

Negative thoughts strengthen in intensity every time you react to them. If you feel angry with your kid and react to the anger by yelling at him or her, or if you throw a huge fit in reaction to something demeaning your sibling said to you, you will only feel more upset, remorseful, and frustrated later.

Reacting to something means you pay heed to the very first irrational thought you experience. To illustrate, if you feel a strong urge to quit your job when your boss does not give you the raise he promised, you may actually quit your job without thinking about the implications of this decision.

Similarly, if you feel upset, you are likely to react to that sadness by holding on to it and overthinking that very emotion. You fixate on it for hours, days, and weeks only to understand its implications when it turns into a chronic emotional problem.

To let go of the negativity, stop reacting to the emotion and **make a conscious effort to respond to it**. Responding to an emotion, a negative thought, or any situation means that you do not engage in the very first reactive thought that pops up in your head, and instead, you take your time to think things through, analyze the situation, and address it from different aspects to make an informed decision. If you carefully respond to your emotions and thoughts that trigger negative behaviors, beliefs, and actions, you will get rid of the negativity in your life and replace it with hope, positivity, and happiness. Here is how you can do that:

- Every time you experience an emotion that stirs up a series of negative thoughts in your head, stop doing the task and recognize the emotion.
- Very carefully and calmly, observe your emotion and let it calm down on its own without reacting to it.
- You need to fight the urges you experience at that time to react to the emotion. Therefore, if you are depressed and keep thinking how terrible you are, and you feel the urge to lock yourself in your room, control it by just staying where you are.
- Give your emotion some time, and it will calm down.
- Try to understand the message it is trying to convey to you. If you are angry with yourself for not qualifying to the next round of an entrepreneurial summit and have lost the chance of winning the grand prize of $1 million, observe your anger and assess it. Ask yourself questions such as: Why do I feel angry? What does the loss mean to me? Asking yourself such questions helps you calm down the strong emotion and let go of the negative thoughts you experience during that time. Naturally, when you stop focusing on the intense emotion and the negative thoughts it triggers, and you divert your attention towards questions to find a way out of the problem, you gently soothe your negative thought process.
- Assess the entire situation in depth and find out ways to better resolve the problem at hand. When you focus on the solution and not the problem, you easily

overcome negative thoughts and create room for possibilities.

It will be difficult to not react to a strong emotion, but if you stay conscious of how you feel and behave, and make consistent efforts, you will slowly nurture the habit to respond to your emotions, which will only help you become more positive.

List of Different emotions

Emotions can usually be categorized into two different types. However, these types come in different forms. Some experts categorize emotions into two types: emotions to be expressed and emotions to be controlled. Others categorize emotions as: primary emotions and secondary emotions. One thing common with both classifications of emotions. However, is all kinds of emotions are usually either positive or negative? Whether an emotion is primary/secondary or expressed/controlled, it will either be negative or positive. Often, people believe that positive psychology is centered mainly on positive emotions but this isn't quite true. In truth, positive psychology leans more towards negative emotions because it is more about managing and overturning negative emotions to achieve positive results.

Firstly, positive emotions may be defined as emotions that provide pleasurable experience; they delight you and do not impact your body unhealthily. Positive emotions, as expected, promote positive self-development. Basically, we are saying that positive emotions are the results of pleasant responses to stimuli in the environment or within ourselves. On the other hand, negative emotions refer to those emotions we do not find particularly pleasant, pleasurable, or delightful to experience. Negative emotions are usually the result of unpleasant responses to stimuli and they cause us to express a negative effect towards a person or a situation.

Naturally, we have different examples of emotions groups under positive and negative. But most times, you can't authoritatively state if emotion is positive or negative. In fact, there are certain emotions that could be both positive and negative. The best way to discern between a positive and negative emotion is to use your intuition. For instance, anger could be both, positive and negative. So, the best way to know when it is negative or when it is positive is to intuitively discern the cause and the context of the anger. This book is, of course, going to focus more on negative emotions and how you can embrace them to create positive results for yourself.

Anger and fear are the two prominent negative emotions which most of us erroneously assume we have to do away with. To be realistic, we cannot allow these emotions to rule our lives yet; we must also understand that they are a necessary part of our experiences as humans. It is impossible to say that you never want to get angry anymore; what is possible is to say that you want to control your anger and get angry less. Mastering negative emotions such as anger is about recognizing and embracing the reality of them, determining their source, and becoming aware of their signs so that we can always know when to expect them and how to control them. For example, if you master an emotion like anger, you naturally start to discern which situation may get you angry and how you could avoid this situation.

A list of negative emotions includes;

- Anger
- Fear
- Anxiety
- Depression

- Sadness

- Grief

- Regret

- Worry

- Guilt

- Pride

- Envy

- Frustration

- Shame

- Denial…and more.

Many people regard negative emotions to be signs of low emotional intelligence or weakness but this aren't right. Negative emotions have a lot of benefits as long as we do not allow them to overrun us. You aren't completely healthy if you do not let out some negative emotions every now and then. One thing you should know is that negative emotions help you consider positive emotions from a counterpoint. If you do not experience negative emotions at all, how then would positive emotions make you feel good? Another thing is that negative emotions are key to our evolution and survival as humans. They direct us to act in ways that are beneficial to our growth, development, and survival as humans. Anger, mostly considered a negative emotion, helps us ascertain and find solutions to problems. Fear teaches us to seek protection from danger; sadness teaches us to find and embrace love and company. It goes on and on like this with every negative emotion there is.

When we talk about negative emotions, we don't actually mean negative as in "bad." The negativity we talk about in relation to certain emotions isn't to portray them as being bad but rather to understand that they lean more towards a negative reality as opposed to positive emotions. Negative emotions, without doubt, can affect our mental and physical state adversely; some primary negative emotions like sadness could result in depression or worry. We must understand that they are designed just for the purpose of making uncomfortable. They could lead to chronic stress when not checked, making us want to escape these emotions. What you should however know is that we cannot completely escape negative emotions; we can only master them so they don't affect us adversely. Often, some of these emotions are geared towards sending us important messages. For example, anxiety may be a telling sign that there is something that needs to be changed and fear may be a sign that a person or situation may endanger our safety.

Overall, what you should know is that these negative emotions you experience aren't something to be gotten rid of. Rather, they are meant to be mastered so we can employ them in achieving the high-functioning, full-of-purpose life that we desire and deserve. Just like positive emotions, negative emotions are meant to protect us and serve as motivation for us to live a better, more qualitative life and build/maintain quality relationships with people around us.

Note: Negative emotions in themselves do not directly have any impact on our mental and physical health and well-being. How we process and react when we experience negative emotions is what actually matters to our health.

Destructive effects of having an anger problem

Have you ever heard of the saying "A thought murder a day keeps the doctor away?" This saying is a quite insightful one which refers to how letting yourself feel angry is a healthy thing to do whereas suppressing or denying feelings of anger can have an immensely pathological effect on you. From past experiences, what we have come to know about anger is that it only becomes destructive to you or people around you when it is repressed or let out unhealthily. Anger can have profoundly negative effects on you, your happiness, and people around you. Suppressing your feelings of anger has consequences which are utterly destructive. When you repress your anger, you have the tendency of becoming psychosomatic which could cause real harm to your body. Holding in your anger creates tension in the body and this may cause stress which is a major player in many of the psychosomatic illnesses which we have. Based on research done in the past, there has been substantial evidence to prove that suppressing anger can be the precursor to cancer development in the body and may also inhibit progress even after the cancer has been diagnosed and is being treated.

There are so many effects anger could have on your health. Let's examine some of these effects.

- **Heart Problems:** Anger puts you at great risk of having a heart attack. The risk of having a heart attack doubles whenever you have an outburst of anger. When you suppress your anger or express it through an unhealthy outlet, the effect goes directly to your heart meaning it could lead to heart problems. In fact, a study has shown that people with anger disorders or volatile anger are more likely to have coronary disease more than people who show less signs of anger. However, constructive or positive anger is in no way related to any heart problem. It could even be very good for your health.

- **Weak Immune System:** Getting angry all the time can actually weaken the immune system, making you prone to more and more illnesses as a study has confirmed. Based on a study conducted in Harvard Medical School, an angry outburst can cause a 6-hour drop in the amount of immunoglobulin A, an antibody responsible for defending the body against infections. Now, imagine if you are always angry; you could really damage your immune system unless you learn to control your anger.

- **Cause Stroke:** You are at a very high risk of having a severe stroke if you are the type who explodes every time. Volatile and habitual anger increases your possibility of developing a stroke ranging from a slightly mild blood clot to the brain to actual bleeding in the brain.

- **Increase Anxiety:** Experiencing anxiety at one point or the other is a normal thing but anger can actually worsen your anxiety if care is not taken. In fact, anger is a primary emotion to anxiety i.e. your anxious feelings may be due to underlying anger problems. Anger increases the symptoms of Generalized Anxiety Disorder (GAD) which is an extreme case of anxiety. People with GAD have higher levels of repressed, internalized, and unexpressed anger which contributes to the development of GAD symptoms; this can be quite destructive.

- **Causes Depression:** Anger increases anxiety which can in turn result in clinical depression. Over the years, many studies have found a link between anger, anxiety, and depression, especially when it comes to men. Passive anger is one of the symptoms of depression; you are constantly angry but too unmotivated to act on the anger.

- **Decreases Lifespan:** Anger results in stress and stress is a very strong suspect when it comes to ill health. Combined with stress, anger can have a really strong effect on your health and it can shorten your lifespan due to the number of health problems it can generate. People who constantly experience repressed anger have shorter lifespans than people who express their anger healthily.

Anger should never be repressed or unhealthily expressed. Instead, you should take active efforts to manage your anger and put it under control so as to avoid all of the negative effects of anger which you have just learned about. Never should you try to stifle or suppress your anger. Suppressing emotions as we have reiterated over the chapters makes it hard to manage them or master them like you should. To start with, pay attention to any feeling of anger you experience and use the information gained to discern where the anger is coming from so that you can use one or more of the anger management techniques we will be checking out below to effectively combat anger problems.

CHAPTER 3: WHAT RULES YOUR EMOTIONS

Emotions can be triggered by all sorts of things from people, places, and times of day or even certain objects. How triggers work is that they activate thoughts or memories in our brain and cause us to have physical and emotional responses.

Having emotions is a normal human reaction to our life circumstances, the problem comes when we are unable to evaluate our emotions or consider their impact on our lives. Most people passively accept their emotions; they don't even get to the points we have covered where they choose to identify what the emotion is or what has triggered it.

How Our Thoughts Shape Our Emotions

During the 1960s, social psychologist Walter Mischel headed several psychological studies on delayed rewards and gratification. He closely studied hundreds of children between the ages of 4 to 5 years to reveal a trait that is known to be one of the most important factors that determine success in a person's life, gratification.

This experiment is famously referred to as the marshmallow test. The experiment involved introducing every child into a private chamber and placing a single marshmallow in front of them. At this stage, the researcher struck a deal with the child.

The researcher informed them that he would be gone from the chamber for a while. The child was then informed that if he or she didn't eat the marshmallow while the researcher was away, he would come back and reward them with an additional marshmallow apart from the one on the table. However, if they did eat the marshmallow placed on the table in front of them, they wouldn't be rewarded with another.

It was clear. One marshmallow immediately or two marshmallows later.

The researcher walked out of the chamber and re-entered after 15 minutes.

Predictably, some children leaped on the marshmallow in front of them and ate it as soon as the researcher walked out of the room. However, others tried hard to restrain themselves by diverting their attention. They bounced, jumped around, and scooted on the chairs to distract themselves in a bid to stop them from eating the marshmallow. However, many of these children failed to resist the temptation and eventually gave in.

Only a handful of children managed to hold until the very end without eating the marshmallow.

The study was published in 1972 and became globally popular as 'The Marshmallow Experiment.' However, it doesn't end here. The real twist in the tale is what followed several years later.

Researchers undertook a follow-up study to track the life and progress of each child who was a part of the initial experiment. They studied several areas of the person's life and were surprised by what they discovered. The children who delayed gratification for higher rewards or waited until the end to earn two marshmallows instead of one had higher school grades, lower instances of substance abuse, lower chances of obesity, and better stress coping abilities.

The research was known as a ground-breaking study on gratification because researchers followed up on the children 40 years after the initial experiment was conducted, and it was sufficiently evident that the group of children who delayed gratification patiently for higher rewards succeeded in all areas they were measured on.

This experiment proved beyond doubt that delaying gratification is one of the most crucial skills for success in life.

Success and delaying gratification

Success usually boils down to picking between the discomfort of discipline over the pleasure and comfort of distraction. This is exactly what delaying gratification is. Would you rather go out for the new movie in town where all your friends are heading, or would you rather sit up and study for an examination to earn good grades? Would you rather party hard with your co-workers before the team gets started with an important upcoming presentation? Or would you sit late and work on fine tuning the presentation?

Our ability to delay gratification is also a huge factor when it comes to decision making and is considered an important aspect of emotional intelligence. Each day, we make several choices and decisions. While some are trivial and have little influence on our future (what color shoes should I buy? Or which way should I take to work?), others have a huge bearing on our success and future.

As human beings, we are wired to make decisions or choices that offer an instant return on investment. We want quick results, actions, and rewards. The mind is naturally tuned for a short-term profit. Why do you think e-commerce giants are making a killing by charging an additional fee for same day and next day delivery? Today is better than tomorrow!

Think about how different our life would be if we thought about the impact of our decisions about three to five years from now? If we can bring about this mental shift where we can delay gratification by keeping our eyes firmly fixated on the bigger picture several years from now, our lives can be very different.

Another factor that is important in gratification delay is the environment. For example, if children who were able to resist temptation were not given a second marshmallow or reward for delaying gratification, they are less likely to view delaying gratification as a positive habit.

If parents do not keep their commitment to reward a child for delaying gratification, the child won't value the trait. Delaying gratification can be picked up only in an environment of commitment and trust, where a second marshmallow is given when deserved.

Examples of gratification delay

Let us say you want to buy your dream car that you see in the showroom on your way to work every day. You imagine how wonderful it would be to own and drive that car. The car costs $25,000, and you barely have $5000 dollars in your current savings. How do you buy the car then? Simple, you start saving. This is how you will combine strong willpower with delayed gratification.

There are countless opportunities for you to blow money every day such as hitting the bar with friends for a drink on weekends, co-workers visiting the nearest coffee shop to grab a latte, or buying expensive gadgets. Every time you remove your wallet to pay, you have two clear choices: either blow your money on monetary pleasure or wait for the long-term reward. If you can resist these temptations and curtail your expenses, you'll be closer to purchasing your dream car. Making this decision will help you buy a highly desirable thing in future.

Will you spend now for immediate gratifications and pleasures, or will you save to buy something more valuable in the future?

Here is another interesting example to elucidate the concept of delayed gratification. Let us say you want to be the best film director the world has ever seen. You want to master the craft and pick up all skills related to movie making and the entertainment business. You visualize yourself as making spectacular movies that inspire and entertain people for decades.

How do you plan to work towards a large goal, or the big picture (well, literally)? You'll start by doing mundane, boring; uninspiring jobs on the sets such as being someone's assistant, fetching them a cup of coffee, cleaning the sets, and other similar boring chores. It isn't exciting or fun, but you go through it each day because you have your eyes firmly fixated on the larger goal, or bigger picture.

You know you want to become a huge filmmaker one day and are prepared to delay gratification for fulfilling that goal. The discomfort of your current life is smaller in comparison to the pleasure of the higher goal. This is delayed gratification. Despite the discomfort, you regulate your actions and behavior for meeting a bigger goal in the future. It may be tough and boring currently, but you know that doing these arduous tasks will give you that shot to make it big someday.

Delayed gratification can be applicable in all aspects of life from health to relationships. Almost every decision we make involves a decision between opting for short-term pleasures now and enjoying bigger rewards later. A burger can give you immediate pleasure today, whereas an apple may not give you instant pleasure but will benefit your body in the long run.

Stop drop technique

Each time you identify an overpowering or stressful emotion that is compelling you to seek immediate pleasure, describe your feelings by writing them down. Make sure you state them clearly to acknowledge their existence.

Have you seen the old VCR models? They had a big pause button prominently placed in the middle. You are now going to push the pause button on your thoughts.

Focus all attention on the heart as it is the center of all your feelings.

Think of something remarkably beautiful that you experienced. It can be a spectacular sunset you witnessed on one of your trips, a beautiful flower you saw in a garden today, or a cute pet kitten you spotted in the neighborhood. Basically, anything that evokes feelings of joy, happiness, and positivity in you. The idea is to bring about a shift in your feelings.

Experience the feeling for some time and allow it to linger. Imagine the feelings you experience in and around your heart. If it is still challenging, take deep breaths. Hold the positive feeling and enjoy it.

Now, click on the mental pause button and revisit the compelling idea that was causing stressful feelings. How does it feel right now?

Now write down how you are feeling and what comes to mind. Act on the fresh insight if it is suitable.

This process doesn't take much time (again, you are craving instant gratification) and makes it easier for you to resist giving in to temptation. The real trick is to change the physical feeling with the heart to bring about a shift in thoughts and eventually, actions. You don't suffocate or undermine your emotions.

Rather, you acknowledge them and then gently change them. When your emotions are slowly changing, the brain tows its line which makes us think in a way that lets us act according to our values and not on impulse or uncontrollable emotions.

Self-mastery is the master key

According to Walter Mischel, "Goal-directed and self-imposed gratification delay is fundamental to the process of emotional self-regulation." Emotional management, or regulation and the ability to control one's impulses, are vital to the concept of emotional intelligence.

Mischel's research established that while some people are born with a greater control for impulses, or better emotional management, others are not. A majority of people are somewhere in between. However, the good news is that emotional management, unlike intelligence, can be learned through practice. EQ isn't as genetically determined as cognitive abilities.

Impulse control and delayed gratification

Have you ever said something in anger and then regretted it immediately? Have you ever acted on an impulse or in haste only to regret it soon after the act? I can't even count the number of people who have lost their jobs, ruined their relationships, nixed their business negotiations, and blown away friendships because of that one moment when they acted on impulse. When you don't allow thoughts to take over and control your words or actions, you demonstrate low emotional intelligence.

Thus, the concept of emotional intelligence is closely connected with delaying gratification. We've all acted at some point or another without worrying about the consequences of our actions. Impulse control, or the ability to construct our thoughts and actions prior to speaking or acting, is a huge part of emotional control. You can manage your emotions more efficiently when you learn to override impulses, which is why impulse control is a huge part of emotional intelligence.

Ever wondered about the reason behind counting to ten, 100, or 1000 before reacting each time you are angry? We've all had our parents and educators counsel us about how anger can be restrained by counting up to ten or 100. It is simple, while you are in the process of counting; your emotional level is slowly decreasing. Once you are done with counting, the overpowering impulse to react to the emotion has passed. This allows you act in a more rational and thoughtful manner.

Emotional intelligence is about identifying these impulsive reactions and regulating them in a more positive and constructive manner. Rather than reacting mindlessly to a situation, you need to stop and think before responding. You choose to respond carefully instead of reacting impulsively to accomplish a more positive outcome or thwart a potentially uncomfortable situation.

Here are some useful tips for delaying gratification and boosting your ability to regulate emotions:

☐ **Have a clear vision for your future**

Delaying gratification and controlling impulses or emotions becomes easier when you have a clear picture of the future. When you know what you want to accomplish five, eight, ten, or 15 years from now, it will be a lot easier to keep the bigger picture in mind if you come across temptations that can ruin your goal. Your 'why' (compelling reason for accomplishing a goal) will keep you sustained throughout the process of meeting the goal. Have a plan to fulfill your goal once you have a clear goal in mind. Identifying your goals and planning how you'll get there will help you resist the temptation more effectively.

☐ **Find ways to distract yourself from temptations and eliminate triggers**

For instance, if you are planning to quit drinking, take a different route back home from work if there are several bars along the way. Instead of focusing on what you can't do, concentrate on the activities you are passionate about. Surround yourself with positive people and activities that will help you dwell on your goal. Avoid trying to fill your time with material goods.

☐ Make spending money difficult

If you are a slave to plastic money and online transactions, you are making the process of spending money too easy for your own good. Paying with cold, hard cash can make you think several times before spending. You'll reconsider your purchases when you pay with real money rather than plastic. Take a part of your salary and put it into a separate account that you won't touch. Make sure that accessing your savings account won't be easy.

☐ Avoid 'all or nothing' thinking

Most of us think resisting temptation or giving up a bad habit is an 'all or nothing challenge.' It is natural for a majority of normal human beings to have a minor slip here and there. However, that doesn't mean you should just fall off and quit. Occasional slip-ups shouldn't be used as an excuse to get off the track. Despite a small detour, you can get back on the track. Don't try to convince yourself to wander in the opposite direction.

☐ Make a list of common rationalizations

Find a counterpoint or counterargument for each. For example, you were angry for just five minutes, or you are spending only ten dollars extra. Tell yourself that five minutes of anger is 150 minutes a month wasted in anger or ten dollars extra is $3,000 extra spent throughout the year.

CHAPTER 4: HOW TO DEAL WITH FEAR, REJECTION, CRITICISM

Anxiety refers to the feeling of uneasiness, fear, or worry that you experience when you encounter a challenge, obstacle, or a nerve-wrecking situation. This feeling is quite natural and normal in situations that demand it. For instance, you are bound to feel nervous when going for a job interview or right before finding out your examination results.

While feeling anxious occasionally or when the need arises is normal, sometimes we tend to hold on to the anxiety for excessively long and to the extent that it becomes engrained in our minds. As a result of this, we feel anxious even when there is no need for it.

How Constant Anxiety Sabotages Our Wellbeing

Feeling extremely apprehensive, pensive, and scared without any solid reason only takes a toll on your mental, emotional, and physical health. You feel scared of taking a step forward worrying it may lead to an unfortunate outcome. You keep thinking of how things will go wrong and stop considering the possibility of things taking a positive turn for once. You doubt your capabilities and incessantly fret over things that may never happen.

This state of constant worry and a racing mind that compels you to imagine the worst-case scenario associated with situations affect every aspect of your life.

- Health: When you keep agonizing over what may happen, you are likely to ignore your health. Often people eat a lot out of stress and anxiety, and this unhealthy eating habit coupled with chronic anxiety paves way for health disorders. Some people also stop eating properly at all when they are anxious - this again is an unhealthy approach towards health and nutrition that only weakens you from within.

- Relationships: If you constantly fuss over things that may never happen, you only waste the precious moments of the present that you could have otherwise spent with your loved ones. Naturally, when you do not spend quality time with loved ones or are always in a state of panic, you stop giving your loved ones the time and energy they need to bond better with you, and this ends up straining your relationships.

- Work Life: Your anxious state of mind directly affects your professional performance. If you remain anxious for days over petty issues, you will only feel distracted while working. This keeps you from attentively working on your projects resulting in frequent errors and low productivity.

- Pursuit of Goals: Naturally, when you are panic-stricken frequently, you don't have the ability and courage to believe in yourself and your goals, and thus, let go of them.

If these problems persist in your life, this only makes life more challenging. While this may be the state of your life, it is not what you want, and if you are sure you wish to live a much better life, it is time you work on overcoming your fears and anxiousness by simply training yourself to better control and manage your emotions.

Here is how you can do that.

Become More Mindful of Your Emotions

You allow your anxiety to increase in intensity and wash you over completely because oftentimes you are not even aware of how you feel. The same applies to all your emotions that lead to unconstructive thoughts that then pave way for problems in your life. Oftentimes, it so happens that you may be doing something physically but are mentally lurking somewhere in the past or future. This state of forgetfulness keeps you from being aware of how and what you feel and triggers your anxiety without you even realizing that.

A good way to thwart this problem is to nurture the state of mindfulness. Mindfulness refers to being completely aware of how you feel without attaching any sort of judgment or label to the feeling. It also encompasses complete consciousness of the environment around you.

When you are mindful of the present moment, you are aware of everything, you feel and experience in that time without worrying about anything else. This enables you to have control of your racing thoughts and the underlying emotions of anxiety and fear easily by bringing back your attention to the present moment.

As you slowly train yourself to live in the moment and not worry about **what may happen**, you overcome your anxiety and fears, one after another and restore peace in your life. Here is how you can nurture the state of complete mindfulness.

- When you are struck with anxiety, acknowledge the emotion you experience and sit with it. Do not identify with it or immerse yourself in the experience. Instead, imagine that you have moved out of your body and are now carefully observing the anxiety from the perspective of the third person. Observe the anxiety carefully and see what it is trying to convey to you. If it brings forth any of your fears, acknowledge it, write it down, and dig deeper into it later to find a solution to the problem. For instance, you may feel anxious of meeting people because you feel they will judge you, and if you dig deeper into this thought, you will realize that it isn't people, but you who are judging yourself. When you become more aware of how you fabricate thoughts that trigger unhealthy emotions, you do not become entangled in such emotions and are able to dissociate yourself from them.

- Every time you work on a task, pay full attention to every step of the process. While washing clothes, observe how the dryer moves and how the clothes spin in the machine. When listening to a presentation by a colleague, pay attention to every word he/she says and keep bringing back your attention to the task at hand every time you wander off in thought. By doing this, you consciously keep yourself focused on the task at hand and let go of any perturbing thoughts that may trigger your anxiety.

- Create a worry period for yourself- a time window wherein you can think of all your worries mindfully. Every time you think of something disturbing, note it down in a journal and remind yourself to reflect on it during the worry period. Keep the worry period limited to 30 to 40 minutes and think of all your problems in that period. Remember to take one concern at a time and then worry about another one, so you deeply analyze it, find the underlying cause, and determine a solution. Also, this makes you more mindful of the problem at hand and keeps you from jumping from one thought to another.

- Apart from doing all of the above, make sure not to put any sort of labels to your emotions because often it is these labels that make us hold on to petty thoughts and create a mountain out of molehill for no particular reason. Your anxiety is neither good nor bad, neither is your happiness. They are both mere emotions. It is only your reaction and response to an emotion that makes it good or bad. Therefore, if you stop reacting to your anxiety by isolating yourself from others and respond to it by slowly facing and overcoming your fears, the same anxiety that you earlier labeled as 'bad' would turn into something more 'positive.' Every time you experience a bout of anxiety or feel scared of something, or experience any other powerful emotion, overcome the urge to tag it with a label. Instead, just observe it and accept it as it is. You will be surprised how the mere act of accepting your emotions calms you down helping you break free of its shackles.

Start by working on any of these techniques and slowly add more to your routine so you build habits of these practices. Consistently working on them will help you nurture a state of mindfulness always, which allows you to track your emotions 24/7.

Take Complete Ownership of Your Feelings

Your feelings are yours to take care of and if you do not take full ownership of them, they are likely to rattle inside you more and make you feel anxious for no solid reason. Every time you feel apprehensive or scared, accept your feelings as they are instead of blaming it on someone else. If you do not feel like going to a social gathering, it is not the fault of the people, but it is your own weakness. If you feel scared of failing in an examination, which is why you don't apply for it, do not take out the anger on your spouse.

Only when you start taking ownership of your feelings are you then able to accept them as your own and positively work towards improving on them. Every time you experience a strong feeling, do not judge yourself based on it and neither blames it on someone else. Instead, write down how and what you feel and accept it fully.

The moment you take accountability of your feelings, you feel a sense of responsibility emerging inside you. This sense of responsibility then enables you to take charge of the situation and do what is right.

Face Your Fears

You can never completely curb your anxiety unless you face the fears it is rooted in. You can only feel strong when you master your emotions of fear and apprehensiveness, and this can only be possible if you actually face that to which you are afraid.

Now that you are aware of how to control your negative thoughts and be mindful of how you feel, consciously make a list of everything that you are afraid of doing. Things such as confronting your feelings to your crush, starting your own business, publishing your book, trying adventure sports, and anything else that you feel is holding you back can go on that list.

Once your list is ready, pick any one fear that you would like to overcome first and create a plan of action to curb it. If you are afraid of speaking publicly but have always wanted to pursue it, prepare a short speech on a topic you are passionate about and practice speaking it for a minute or two in front of the mirror.

Once you have command over it, speak on the topic in front of 2 to 3 people. You may stumble and make mistakes, but if you do manage to stay strong in that time, you will overcome a part of your fear. Slowly keep speaking in front of more people and soon enough, you will have overcome your fear.

After overcoming one little fear, take on another one, and then another one. Keep combatting your fears this way and thwart them one after another to have better control of your emotions and master them. Remember to record your daily activities and performance in a journal so that you can go through the accounts time and again. This gives insight into your strengths, mistakes, setbacks and accomplishments so that you feel motivated on acknowledging your accomplishments, learn from your mistakes, and improve on them to only do better the next time.

CHAPTER 5: HOW TO DEAL WITH NEGATIVE PEOPLE

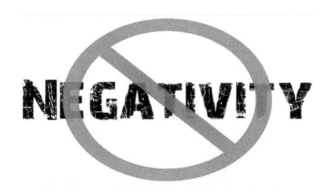

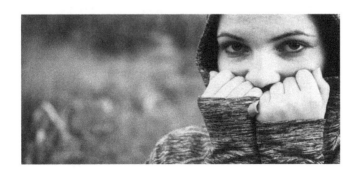

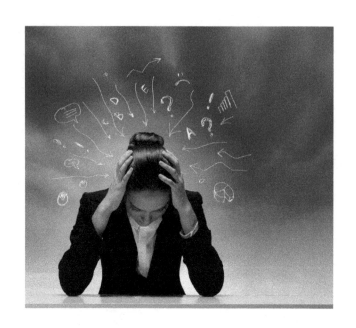

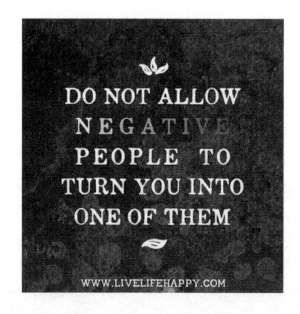

DO NOT ALLOW
NEGATIVE
PEOPLE TO
TURN YOU INTO
ONE OF THEM

WWW.LIVELIFEHAPPY.COM

People as social beings are influenced by what they hear, what they see, what they smell, what they taste and by what they feel. Therefore, other people automatically always have some influence on you. But what happens if this influence is (constantly) negative? You become passive, depressed and frustrated.

If you have negative people around you, you should still be as positive as possible and not let yourself become infected.

If someone (again) complains about the bad weather, you should not start a discussion with them or try to convince them, but rather change the subject, if possible, towards something that interests them or is their passion.

Another way to deal with negative people is to clearly express your opinion: "I cannot stand your whining and your negativity anymore. You therefore have two options in my presence. Either you are silent or one of us is leaving." You need self-confidence in order to do this and this approach does not work with everyone. But there are some people with whom it works wonderfully to put a mirror in front of their face, because they have never really reflected themselves and been shown how much they play the victim.

If you feel like you are surrounded by negative people it might also be because of yourself, as tough as that sounds. Because usually we attract people who are like us.

Based on the quote above you should always remember that it is easier to change your environment than to change the people around you. You can achieve this successfully if you separate yourself spatially from your previous environment as well and build yourself a new identity in a previously unknown place where nobody knows you. Because then you can choose yourself who you allow to become part of your life and from the very beginning you can allow positive people into your life and avoid negative people and surround you with an environment that is good for you. This may be a drastic measure for some and does not seem easy to implement, but it leads to the desired goal more effectively and faster. Because you cannot change people who all have their own life stories, traits and habits that distinguish them, as long as they do not want that change themselves. Surround yourself with people who give you a positive feeling, who help you, from whom you can learn something, because they are further developed than you. Think well with whom to share your valuable lifetime.

How you can stop negative feelings and thoughts!

Here are 5 tips on how to effectively deal with negative feelings and thoughts:

Tip 1

Imagine your negative thoughts are like clouds. Just because you can see them does not necessarily mean you need to identify with them. They are there but they will disappear again. It is the same with your negative feelings. Instead of saying you are sad, you could tell yourself something inside of you is sad. That is how you create a certain distance and you do not identify so strongly with your thoughts and feelings.

Tip 2

Write down your negative thoughts and feelings as they occur. Try to put into words what you think and what you feel. That also means writing down questions about where these thoughts might come from. Keep writing until you cannot think of anything else and you will realize it will then be much easier for you to better organize and process your thoughts and feelings. You will gain more clarity.

Tip 3

Breathe deeply and consciously. Because your breath is the enemy of your negative thoughts. When you breathe and just accept that your negative feelings are there you relax. And once you relax, you no longer fight against your emotional state, making it easier for those feelings to disappear.

Tip 4

Whenever negative thoughts and feelings appear remember you are mortal. The very idea that one could theoretically die the next day sets the current emotional state of a person in relation to the worst case that could occur. This usually leads to the doubt whether what you think or feel at the time is really as crucial as you might think? In other words: the negative thought is put in relation to a much worse scenario and thus does not appear as large as before.

Tip 5

If you have concrete goals in your life and follow your passion constantly making new achievements you are effectively countering the negative spiral. As you begin to value and use your precious time more effectively, the space for negative thoughts becomes smaller and smaller. Start acting instead of stopping. To take action is a constant process that can be imagined as clean, flowing water. Stagnant water begins to stink after a while due to the spreading of putrefactive bacteria. So plan your day and follow specific goals in your life that you work on daily. This puts your focus back on things that work and give you a sense of success and satisfaction.

CONCLUSION

Emotions are predominantly sited in the unconscious implying that we have significantly less control of how emotions occur. It is for this reason, that body language is critical in determining the true status of an individual as the unconscious impacts much of the body language. With all these developments, emotions are highly manageable. The book emphasized consistently that the focus should not be on preventing emotions but allowing them to manifest safely. Most people have the wrong assumption that negative emotions should not be expressed forgetting that emotions are a form of energy, and they need to dissipate.

Your emotions are here to guide you. Learn as much as you can from them, and then let them go. Don't cling to them as if your existence depends on them. It doesn't. Don't identify with them as though they define you. They don't. Instead, use your emotions to grow and remember, you are beyond emotions.

Lightning Source UK Ltd.
Milton Keynes UK
UKHW020641100521
383461UK00014B/914